The Fiber Cleanse

A Research-Based Detox Diet That Will Improve Overall Health and Promote Weight Loss

Christopher P. Doyle

Table of Contents

Introduction

If you have been on a weight-loss or general healthy living journey for any number of years, I'm sure you have come across countless diets and detoxes. Many of these are just fad diets that have no real evidence behind them but instead promote fast weight loss. When something promises extreme weight loss in a short period of time, it is usually unsustainable and unhealthy.

Many of these diets leave out important food groups and that means your body is not getting all the nutrients it needs to function properly. Juice cleanses are a popular 'detox' that many people are trying; however, there is no lasting benefit to doing this. Even diets like keto and the Atkins diet cut out important food groups. Naturally, if you are not eating a specific food group, you will lose weight because you are eating less. The problem is that as soon as you want to go back to eating normally, you will gain all that weight back, and most often, even more!

Eating is meant to be an enjoyable experience, but unfortunately, all these overly restrictive diets and detoxes cause us to have a negative view of and relationship with food. The chances of you binge eating after trying these methods are extremely high. This leaves people feeling even worse about themselves than they did before.

The best diets are those that are sustainable and do not limit you by cutting out large food groups. You still need to have a balanced diet; our bodies need a blanched amount of fats, proteins, and carbohydrates. If you get this right, you will have a healthy nutritional balance and feel so much better about yourself.

One of the most important elements to a healthy diet that often gets overlooked is fiber. Not many people are aware of the benefits of fiber in their bodies and the foods that are easily available are usually not fiber dense. Getting enough fiber in our diets should be a priority for everyone, whether you want to lose weight or just be healthier.

Foods rich in fiber are much healthier for you and will help you have a balanced diet and receive increased health benefits. Throughout this book, we will go through what fiber is and how to add more of it into your diet. When you do this, you will be able to facilitate successful weight loss, lead a healthier life, ward off certain diseases, and reap the many other benefits fiber has to offer.

Chapter 1: What Is Fiber?

Most of us have been given the advice to "eat more fiber." If you are like me, you have probably brushed it off without much thought. The truth is that this is great advice we should all be taking. However, it makes it hard to understand why if we don't have a good knowledge of fiber, what it is, and where to get it from.

Insoluble vs. Soluble Fiber

Fiber is the part of food that is not able to be digested; instead, it just passes through your body in a relatively whole form (Mayo Clinic, 2018c). Dietary fiber can be classified as a carbohydrate; the difference between fiber and other carbohydrates is that fiber is not broken down into sugars and stored. Fiber can be broken up into two categories, each have their own benefits and react in the body in a different way. These categories are insoluble and soluble fiber; they can both be found in plant sources but the amount of each will vary.

Insoluble fiber is the type of fiber that is referred to when speaking about bowel movements. It increases the regularity and bulk of stool, making it easier to pass out of the system. It isn't dissolved by water or broken down by the body. Since it passes through the digestive tract without being absorbed, it is not a source of calories. This does not mean that the foods in which you find insoluble fiber is calorie free (Butler, 2017). Fiber just makes up a part of the food, but in general, foods high in insoluble fiber are lower in calories.

Soluble fiber, unlike insoluble fiber, dissolves in water and turns into a gel-like substance (Mayo Clinic, 2018c). It is then digested by bacteria in the gut, and because of this process, it does release some calories. When you eat foods high in soluble fiber, you will feel fuller for longer because it slows down the pace of digestion as it takes up a large space in your stomach.

Where Can I Find Fiber?

Now that you understand the basics of fiber, you can add it to your diet. You will want to add the right foods to get a good amount of fiber into your body every day. Dietary fiber is found in many plants and whole foods. In general, whole grains, fruit, vegetables, beans, legumes, nuts, and seeds are all good sources of fiber. High fiber is called "roughage'" for a reason; anything that has been processed to a point of being quite smooth probably does not have a lot of fiber. Think about the difference in texture and taste with whole wheat bread and white bread.

When it comes to eating fruit and vegetables, after washing thoroughly, leave the skins on, where you will find the most fiber. Of course, there are some cases where you cannot eat the skins; oranges and pumpkin can be peeled. Apples, pears, and cucumbers are good examples that can be eaten with the skin on.

The more processed the food, the less fiber it will have. This includes enriched foods; usually, some vitamins are added back but not the fiber. If you are looking to get a high fiber diet, you should stay away from most processed foods. When the food is processed, the husks are removed and this is the part that contains the fiber. This is also the problem with a lot of juice cleanses: all the fiber is removed from the fruit and vegetables and you miss all the benefits.

If you do eat a lot of packaged or processed foods, then you can look at labels on food packages to see how much fiber is in the product. If the label says it is high in fiber, then it should contain at least 20% of the recommended daily amount of fiber; foods that are lower than 5% fiber are considered low in fiber, according to the guidelines set out by the FDA (Butler, 2017). There are a lot of high fiber options, but you will have to make an effort to look for them. There tends to be a higher amount of low fiber processed foods than high fiber foods available at supermarkets.

You should be aiming to get a good amount of both insoluble and soluble fiber. Soluble fiber can be found in foods like broccoli, black beans, lima beans, turnips, brussels sprouts, avocado, sweet potato, and pears. Insoluble fiber can be found in foods like whole wheat flour, wheat bran, cauliflower, green beans, and regular potatoes (McManus, 2019). Adding these foods to your diet will boost your fiber intake and allow you to reap the many benefits of a fiber rich diet.

Chapter 2: The Many Benefits of Fiber

We have spoken about fiber passing through your system, but don't think that it does so idly. Fiber performs many functions as it moves through our bodies; it is definitely put to work through its journey. As you go through this chapter, you will see why you should always be getting enough fiber in your diet.

A Breakdown of the Benefits

Fiber is so good for us as it provides so many benefits. This is probably why it is available in so many foods. In order to understand why we should eat a high-fiber diet, we need to know the benefits of following such a diet or adding more fiber to the eating plan we already follow.

Normalizes Bowel Movements

Constipation is a common problem many people suffer from. It most certainly has to do with what you eat. High-fiber diets reduce the risk of constipation because the fiber will add some bulk to the stool, and bulkier stool is easier to pass. If you have the opposite problem, where you have stool that is very loose, fiber will help remedy this as well. The fiber will stiffen up the stool by absorbing liquids and this will result in an easier and more regulated bowel movement.

Assists in Maintaining Bowel Health

A healthy bowel equals a healthy life and it all starts with what we put into our bodies. There have been many studies done on the effects of fiber in the gut and the results come out positive. A high-fiber diet has been shown to reduce the risk of colorectal cancer, hemorrhoids, and developing small pouches in your colon called diverticular disease (Mayo Clinic, 2018c).

Fiber also helps foster healthy gut bacteria. When fiber enters your system, some of it is left behind and ferments in the gut; this creates the perfect living conditions for these bacteria. Through this process, short-chain fatty acids are produced and this has a whole host of benefits including lowering systemic inflammation, which has been linked to many chronic health problems (Dreisbach, n.d.).

Lowers Cholesterol Levels

Fiber, in general, has many benefits, but soluble and insoluble fiber can have different benefits. Soluble fiber is known to reduce cholesterol levels; high cholesterol is linked to heart problems. Of course, a certain amount of cholesterol is needed in our body to perform certain bodily functions, but the problem comes when there is too much cholesterol and this build-up leads to heart problems and other negative effects. As the soluble fiber moves through the body, it grabs the excess fats and cholesterol; this stops it from being absorbed into the bloodstream (Matala, 2018). The fats and cholesterol are then passed out with the fiber. Oats are an extremely good food for doing this; if you do suffer from high cholesterol, then adding some oats to your daily diet can dramatically lower your cholesterol levels.

Heart Health Benefits

Studies have shown that increasing your fiber intake by seven grams per day can lower your risk of heart disease by about 9% (Dreisbach, n.d.). Many heart problems are caused by high blood pressure, or hypertension, which puts unnecessary pressure on the heart and arteries. Fruit and vegetables rich in fiber also contain phytonutrients, which protect the heart by keeping the arteries nice and flexible, as well as keeping the blood flowing at an optimal pace (Agatston, 2009). Anything that helps regulate blood flow and protect the arteries will also, by default, be good for the heart.

Helps Control Blood Sugar

Fiber can help control and regulate your blood sugar. This is done by slowing down digestion of starches and sugars; when this happens, it prevents blood sugar spikes. Our blood sugar spikes up when we eat and is heightened when we eat certain foods. These spikes are not good for us and can cause us to have high levels of energy and then suddenly crash afterwards. Starches and sugars are truly the culprit for blood sugar spikes, and when we have a spike, we then crave more sugars and starches, thus creating a cycle. It is best to curb this and maintain a stable blood pressure.

Assists in Achieving and Maintaining a Healthy Weight

It is common knowledge that when we feel hungry, we eat; however, there are some foods that make us feel hungry quicker and those that fill us up for longer. Foods high in starches and sugars usually make us feel satisfied for a short while, then we will get hungry again and crave more starches and sugars. These foods are also much higher in calories than foods high in fiber. Eating these types of foods can quickly lead to weight gain.

On the other hand, eating foods high in fiber will keep you fuller for longer and do not result in any cravings that could cause you to eat unnecessarily. High fiber foods give you good value for the calories you are eating, so you can eat less and still be full. This is due to the fact that it takes longer for your body to digest fiber than most other foods.

Linked to a Lower Risk of Cardiovascular Disease and Cancer

With all the benefits that fiber has, it also has been linked to reducing the risk of a few other diseases. Studies are still being done to confirm why this is, but a study funded by the National Cancer Institute reported that people who have a high amount of fiber in their diet have the lowest incidence of colon polyps (Agatston, 2009). There is continuous studies on this topic, but there is definitely a correlation between a lower risk of certain diseases and a high fiber diet.

Chapter 3: A Fiber Deficient World

In today's society, there has not been much emphasis put on the importance of fiber. In fact, we don't hear about it all that often. Many people are not even aware of what foods contain fiber and which do not. We are going to go through a few different aspects of living in a fiber deficit world and what it is doing to our bodies.

How Much Fiber Do We Need?

We all need a good amount of fiber in our bodies for us to reap all the benefits it gives. The daily recommended amount of fiber for an adult male under the age of 50 is 38 grams, for a female in the same age group it is 25 grams (McManus, 2019). So, now that we know how much we should be getting, we need to ensure we are getting enough. The average American only gets about 10 to 15 grams of fiber per day; that is less than half the recommended amount. If you were wondering why there are so many health problems in America, this could be a huge contributor.

It can be quite easy to track the amount of fiber you are getting but you don't need to track everything you put into your mouth. Consciously adding foods that are naturally high in fiber and making the right food swaps will easily increase your fiber intake. Natural sources and whole grains are the best options; sometimes labels on packaging can be misleading. Don't just believe that something is high in fiber if it says 'multi-grain' on the packaging; look at the nutritional information on the back. This will give you a better indication of what is in your food.

When looking at the label, if it has the word 'whole' as the first word in the ingredient list, then it may likely have a good amount of fiber in it. Whole grains substitutes are available for pasta, bread, rolls, rice, and most other starches. You don't need to give up your bread and rice if you make the swap; this is probably the easiest way to increase your fiber intake and get the recommended amount of fiber each day. These whole grain foods also add a lovely texture and nutty flavor to your food for an increased flavor profile.

Why Aren't We Getting Enough Fiber?

Many of the foods we are eating are very low in fiber because they are overly processed. If we look at the foods that are readily available to us, we can quickly see they are not whole foods. The convenience of unhealthy, low fiber foods is definitely a big contributor to lower fiber intake of most people. Fast food restaurants mostly serve low fiber foods and usually don't have whole grain, fresh options; this means when we are in need of a quick meal, we will not be getting the fiber we need from it.

Whole foods do require some sort of effort because they are fresher, so fruit and vegetables will go bad if you leave them for too long, whereas other more convenient foods and snacks can be stored for long periods of time and just pulled out of the package to be eaten. When it comes to whole grain starches, these can seem less available than white starches, so they can be missed in the store. If you take a look, you will easily find them on the shelves; they are probably not promoted as much but they are available in most stores.

There is also not enough emphasis placed on fiber and its importance. Most people are just not aware of fiber and the role it plays in the body, so it is up to us to become aware of fiber and how it affects our body. Now that you are aware of fiber and its benefits, you will be more motivated to add it into your diet and will be able to recognize what foods are high in fiber and which are not.

Negative Effects From Lack of Fiber

We have already spoken about the benefits from a high-fiber diet, but there are also negative effects from getting too little fiber in your diet. In fact, you will be able to easily see if you do not get enough fiber because your body will tell you; all you have to do is recognize the signs. Most of the time our body will signal us when it needs something but we just haven't been trained to notice it.

I will mention the most common side effects but there might be others; everyone's bodies are different. If you suspect you are in a fiber deficit, then try and add in more fiber to your diet and see if the symptoms you are experiencing subside. You should always check with your dietician before making any drastic changes to your diet as they would be able to guide you using your specific needs.

Irregular Bowel Movements

Irregular bowel movements can be in the form of constipation or soft stools. Both of these problems can be a result of not having enough fiber in your diet. Fiber helps bowels move smoothly through the system. It adds bulk and firms it up if you are suffering from loose stools. You should be having at least three bowel movements every week. This is recommended for a healthy digestive tract.

Constipation can be caused by other things, such as taking iron and certain other medications. So, be aware of this before you assume that it is a fiber issue; no matter how much fiber you eat, you might still be constipated if it is caused by medication. This can be discussed with your doctor. If there isn't another cause for the constipation, then eating fiber rich foods will most likely help solve that problem.

Weight Gain

As we have discussed before, high fiber foods make you feel fuller for longer. This means that you will not have to eat as much and have a lesser chance of eating unhealthy foods. If you are gaining weight, you should have a look at your diet. Is it filled with processed and preserved foods? If so, this could be the cause of your weight gain.

It is not necessarily cutting out all other foods but increasing fiber intake. Once you start eating more fiber, you will naturally not want to eat so much of the other foods that may not be as good for you. In general, if you are experiencing weight gain, diet is the main factor, and a fiber rich diet can be a turning point.

Fluctuation in Blood Sugar

If you are struggling with controlling your blood pressure, then this can be an indication of you not getting enough fiber. Many diabetics are advised to get more fiber to counteract this. If you are diabetic and are noticing spikes and drop in blood sugar levels, speak to your doctor as this could be linked to low fiber consumption. The fiber will help absorb the sugar in your body and stabilize your blood sugar levels.

Tiredness or Nausea

Tiredness and nausea can be an indication of many things, but if you are experiencing this with one of the other mentioned symptoms, then low fiber might be to blame. High fat and protein diets that are not balanced with high fiber carbohydrates can lead to high cholesterol and fat levels. This could make you feel tired, nauseous, or even weak. Try adding a few more grams of fiber into your meals and remove foods that are high in fat. If these feelings continue, then please consult with a doctor who will be able to point you in the right direction.

Disrupts the Gut's Microbiome

Living in our gut are millions of bacteria of different kinds; these bacteria are what help us digest food and keep our digestive tract healthy. These are all good bacteria and they feed on fiber. If we do not have enough fiber in our diet, these bacteria have nothing to feed on so they start diminishing. The less of them we have, the less healthy we become; this is because these good bacteria protect the gut from bad bacteria.

It's not hard to imagine that the bad bacteria are what causes us to feel sick and can cause a whole host of other problems. Some of the problems these harmful bacteria cause are obesity and inflammatory bowel disease. The best thing we can do is keep our gut microbiome flourishing by eating enough fiber so the good bacteria can thrive and protect the digestive tract.

Lack of Energy

Diets that are high in fat and protein but lacking carbohydrates can leave you feeling as though your energy source is depleted. Our bodies burn carbohydrates for energy, and when they are high fiber carbohydrates, it burns slower for a consistent production of energy.

We obviously need energy throughout the day and when we don't get it from the right sources, our bodies crave a quick fix in sugary foods. When carbohydrates are burned, they are turned into sugars for the body to use as energy. These are good sugars because they are natural and not refined. However, this is the reason our bodies crave sugary foods when we don't have enough energy; unfortunately most of the sugars we crave are

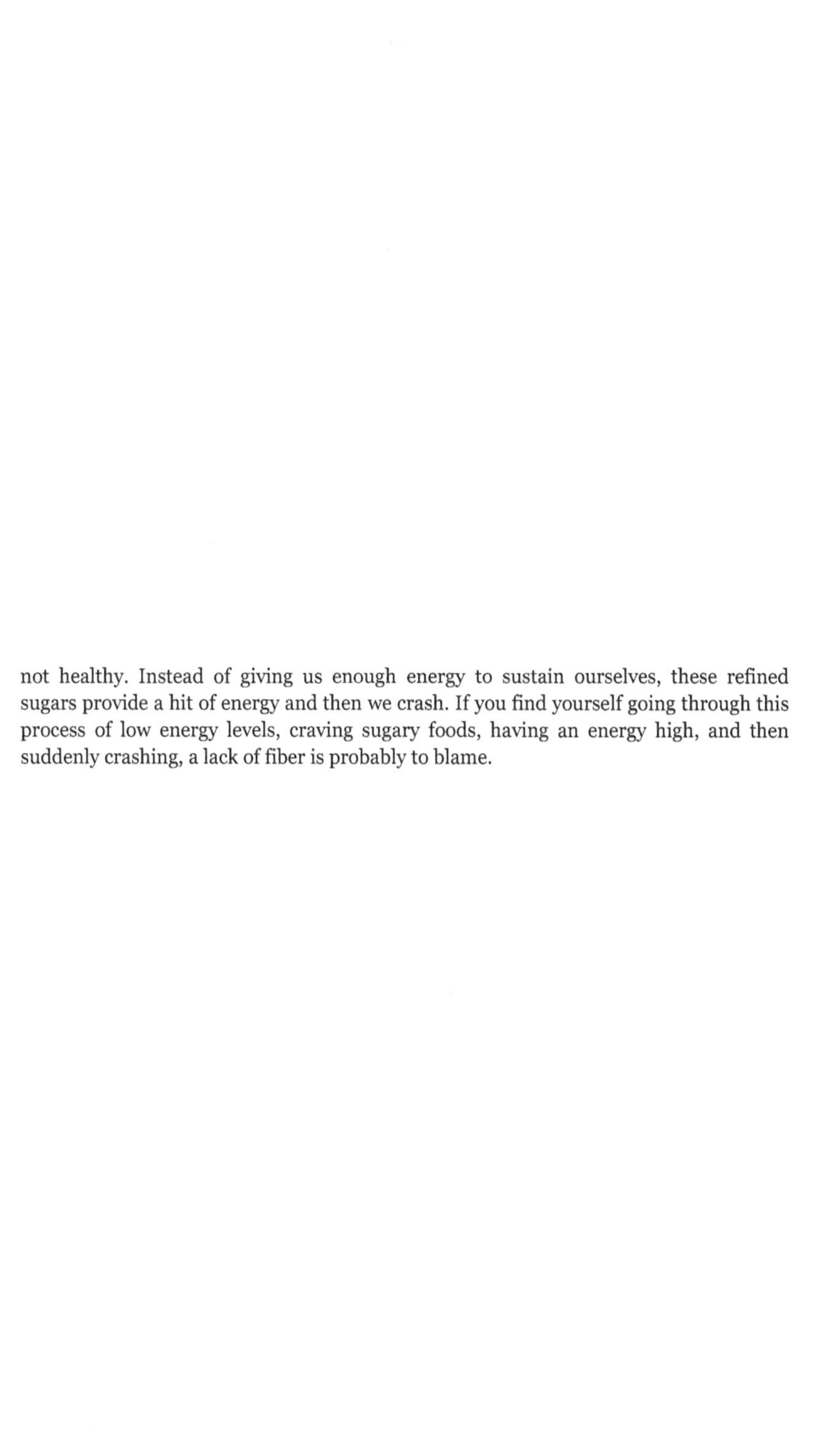

not healthy. Instead of giving us enough energy to sustain ourselves, these refined sugars provide a hit of energy and then we crash. If you find yourself going through this process of low energy levels, craving sugary foods, having an energy high, and then suddenly crashing, a lack of fiber is probably to blame.

Chapter 4: Introduction to the Fiber Cleanse

The fiber cleanse is not another quick detox but rather a shift in lifestyle. Our bodies constantly need to be cleansed from the things we put in it, so it makes sense to add something to our daily life rather than just doing something in the moment. In any case, it is always better to do things the natural way than adding in something that is artificial or that your body would just not come across in normal situations.

What Is a Fiber Cleanse?

A fiber cleanse is just a way to add in extra fiber into your diet so your body will be able to clean itself out. This cleanse creates an environment for good colon health and allows your digestive tract to perform at its best. Unlike other cleanses and detoxes, this does not just last a short while; if you implement it into your life, your body will always be cleaning itself out, and this will lead to a healthier body over time.

Another problem with quick detoxes and cleanses is that there really isn't much scientific evidence to back it up. There have been a few studies done here and there but much of the research is spotty and not definitive. The benefits of a high-fiber diet coupled with enough water has been scientifically proven to help with weight loss and there is very little, if anything, said to dispute it.

A fiber cleanse is not about taking something away from your body but adding something in that your body needs. Our bodies were designed to be self-cleansing; they just need a little help from the food we eat. All you have to do to take part in a fiber cleanse is increase the amount of fiber to a healthy amount and then make sure you are getting enough water, since fiber absorbs liquid. The fiber will help you to not consume unhealthy foods since you will already feel full and it will help eliminate anything that your body does not need.

Our bodies already know what is not good for it and what it needs to function optimally. That is why we have the excretory process. If we eat unhealthy low fiber foods, it makes it harder for the body to eliminate the toxins and unwanted waste, so it just sits in our colon and can cause problems for us. Eating fiber does not change the processes in our bodies but just helps it along when it needs it. That is the premise of a fiber cleanse.

The Fiber Cleanse and Your Digestive Tract

The digestive system is a series of organs that all work together to consume, digest, and eliminate food in our bodies. It consists of the mouth, esophagus, stomach, small intestine, large intestine, and anus, but there are other organs also involved such as the tongue, pancreas, and liver (Bodian, 2019). Food is broken down and all the nutrients the body needs is pulled out of the food; whatever is left is eliminated from the body. This process is vital for the body to function; without the necessary nutrients, we would have no energy and our bodies would essentially wither away.

The digestive tract is such a vital part of the body, but it often gets overlooked. In many cases, if we are not feeling well, it could be a result of something in our digestive tract not agreeing with us, or perhaps it is simply not functioning at optimal efficiency. We want our digestive system to be healthy and functioning properly since it is a vital part of our everyday life.

A fiber cleanse and just eating fiber in general is so good for the colon and the rest of the digestive tract because it basically sweeps it clean. The insoluble fiber bulks up everything in your colon; it is basically gathering up whatever is not needed by the body in order to remove it. The soluble fiber that forms a gel-like substance makes the stool easier to pass. As a result of these working together, you get a completely clean colon and digestive tract.

The above process means there is very little chance of something being left behind in the colon. Anything left in the colon for too long could result in you feeling very uncomfortable and your body not being able to function at 100%.

Not only is a clean colon important but a strong and healthy one is as well. The addition of vitamin D3 and calcium to your diet can actually help prevent colon cancer (Brusie & Cirino, 2017). This is done by preventing inflammation and limiting the chemicals that can cause the cancer to grow and spread. You can find calcium and vitamin D3 in dark leafy green vegetables, dairy produce, and certain fortified cereals. Two of these three are high in fiber as well, so that is a bonus.

Tips to Add More Fiber Into Your Diet

The main goal of having a high-fiber diet is to increase your fiber intake but to also make sure that it turns into a lifestyle and not just a quick fix. If it is going to turn into a lifestyle, it should be relatively easy to integrate fiber into your everyday life and be easy to sustain. The tips below should help you with this and help you be successful in this process.

Meat-Free Mondays

You have probably heard of this term before. Originally, it was used to help people eat less meat since it can be bad for the planet; however, it will also help with increasing fiber intake. It is not that meat is bad or that we want to cut it out completely; it just doesn't have a lot of fiber in it. We can rather replace it with something that is just as filling but has much more fiber in it.

Think about your meals. It might be easier to swap out some meat for veggies. Instead of having a chili made with minced meat, opt for beans, mushrooms, and zucchini. It is still delicious but it has a lot more fiber in it. You could also try swapping out meat for chickpeas or lentils; both of these are filled with protein and fiber to keep you filled up. Doing this once a week for a whole day or even just having one meat-free meal a day will significantly up your fiber intake.

Add Fiber Into Every Meal

You might get fed up with eating fiber if you choose to just pump it all into one sitting; rather, break it up amongst your meals for the day. Spreading it out will allow you to get a variety of high fiber foods throughout the day. You will have less of a chance of getting bored with what you are eating.

Another benefit of this is that you will be able to keep your energy up throughout the day. The fiber will continuously and slowly release energy for you to use, so you don't have to worry about hitting an energy crash. It will also help you eat less at meals; naturally, food with lots of fiber requires more chewing. This gives your body time to register that you are full and you can stop overeating.

When we eat too fast, we often only realize we are full after we are done and then we feel completely stuffed. There is a delayed reaction between the stomach and the brain, so we need to account for that. In general, the slower you eat, the less you will end up eating because it gives our bodies time to catch up with how we are feeling. Instead of leaving the meal completely stuffed, you will be satisfied and won't feel that after meal slump.

Add Your Own Ingredients

Many recipes can be tweaked just a little to bring up the fiber content; there is no rule that states you have to follow the recipe. If you are making your favorite pasta dish, why not add in some broccoli, spinach, or even some peas. You can add beans or nuts to salads. Try blitzing up some chickpeas and adding it as a spread to your favorite lunch time sandwich.

Adding your own spin to these meals will allow you to add in more fiber, get in some different flavors, and get a little creative. Sometimes, it's not about reworking your whole eating plan but rather finding ways to better what you are already eating. Who knows, perhaps you will end up making a new family favorite?

Snack on Fruit and Vegetables

Fruit and vegetables are very high in fiber compared to other snacks; not only that, but they are low in calories and are nutrient dense. They make the perfect snack that is both healthy and will fill you up. You can eat them as is or add a dip.

There are lots of vegetables to choose from; meal prepping them for the week makes it convenient for you to just grab when you are feeling for a snack. Chop up celery, carrots, green beans, and whatever else you want, place them in the fridge, and you can submerge them in water to keep for longer. Grab a few when you need a snack, and serve it with a side of hummus. The chickpeas in hummus are also a good source of fiber.

Soups

Perhaps you are not a fan of the texture of some of the foods or would like something to make in bulk. Soups are your best bet. You can add many vegetables in a soup and you can make it a smooth soup or a more textured one by leaving some of the vegetables whole or roughly chopped. Making soup in a big batch and then freezing it saves you a lot of time and it is an easy lunch or dinner meal on very busy days. There is no need to skip out on your fiber if you have something at the ready.

Start the Day off With Fiber

Cereals can be some of the biggest sources of fiber. If your breakfast is filled with fiber, you won't be as hungry throughout the day and you will find your energy lasts longer. Bran cereals are the highest in fiber; some contain about 10 to 12 grams of fiber per serving. If you pair that with a fruit, like an apple or an orange, then you have already got half of your fiber for the day.

These cereals fill you up but won't make you feel like you have overdone it with the fiber. Bran flakes and variations of that are great options for you. Oats are also a great high fiber breakfast food; they usually contain about half the fiber of bran cereals but still have a significant amount. Oats will leave you feeling full for a long period of time.

Try Chia Seeds

Recently, chia seeds have gained popularity as a superfood. A superfood is one that has lots of benefits and contains various vitamins and minerals; in short, they are very good for you. Not only do they have all of the above benefits but they are also full of fiber. Chia seeds can be easily added to anything since they do not have a strong flavor; instead, they soak up whatever they are put in.

Using chia seeds to make chia pudding has become very popular; all you have to do is add a few spoons of the seeds to a glass of milk, add in your flavoring, and let it sit overnight. When you come back, the chia seeds will have soaked up all the liquid and you are left with a pudding-like dessert. You can also add them on top of oats, in smoothies, in eggs, and anything else you can think of.

Bulgur and Quinoa to Salads

Bulgur and quinoa are both great sources of fiber and they are also quite versatile. If you are lacking fiber in your diet, try swapping out your rice or other grains with either of these two. It's not that (brown) rice is not high in fiber, but bulgur and quinoa are much more so. You can also add them to salads; they add texture and flavor to a plain salad.

Most people miss out on how versatile they are because they haven't tried them in a salad. They are small enough, so they stick to the salad vegetables and can be eaten warm or cold. You can also add them to your mixed roast vegetables for the warm salad option. They both soak up the juices and flavor of the liquid they are cooked in, so you can just add in some stock, broth, or whatever you are cooking with in the moment to make the dish even tastier.

Bake With Alternative Flour

If you are an avid baker, then why not swap out your regular, refined, white flour for a flour that has a much higher fiber content. Luckily, you can now get many different types of flours, so you are free to pick whichever one suits your tastes. You can go for something simple like plain whole wheat flour or you can try coconut, almond, soy, chickpea, buckwheat, or barley flour.

Most of these flours give a similar texture to the regular white flour but it depends on how much you use and the type of baked goods you are making. Most of it will be trial and error but you can also do a search for recipes using alternative flours; there will be plenty to choose from on the internet and most have reviews from people who have already tried it.

Can You Have Too Much Fiber?

We have been discussing the benefits of adding fiber to your diet but this wouldn't be a balanced book if we didn't talk about the possible negative side effects of fiber. Fiber is generally good on all fronts; the only time you might experience something negative is if you have had an excessive amount of it. Too much of a good thing can turn out bad.

We know that fiber is used to pick up toxins and soak up liquids; too much fiber can cause certain nutrient deficiencies because of this same reason. Fiber binds with minerals, some of which are calcium, magnesium, zinc, and iron (Olsen, 2018). The threshold here is when you are eating over 70 grams of fiber in a day, this is way over the daily recommendation for both men and women.

It might seem as if it would be impossible to eat that much fiber in a day, but it can easily happen if you are obsessively adding in fiber to your diet. Eating nutrition bars that have a high fiber content and foods that have extra fiber added in can all quickly add up and push you over the limit. Even though fiber is really good for you, don't try and eat so much of it that you get to a point where it is excessive.

There are symptoms of too much fiber; if you notice you have a few, then take a step back to look at your diet. You may have to cut back on the amount of fiber you are putting into your body. Some of the side effects are bloating, gas, dehydration, stomach cramps, weight gain or weight loss, and nausea. This can be an uncomfortable experience; if you are still experiencing these symptoms and you have tried reducing your fiber intake, then it would be wise to seek the advice of a medical professional. Some of these symptoms are similar to those you would experience with too little fiber in your system, so you will have to take a look at what you have been eating before reducing the amount of fiber you are putting into your body.

There are a few things you can do besides limiting fiber consumption to help your body relieve the symptoms of too much fiber. Fiber absorbs liquid and that is why you might feel dehydrated; to counteract this, you will need to drink more water. Make sure you are getting the recommended amount of water for your weight and you may drink a little more if necessary. Exercise more; this will aid your body in getting the blood flowing to your digestive system. Also, remember to avoid any foods that let air into your stomach; this includes sodas and chewing gum.

If you really have severe symptoms, then you may have to eat a very low fiber diet until the symptoms disappear. A low fiber diet will be about 10 grams or less. Try going for more protein-heavy foods than foods with high carbohydrate levels. Meats and items made with white refined flours are good options. Just remember that this is a temporary diet plan and you will need to bring your fiber intake back up once the symptoms subside; this time stick to the recommended amount of fiber and try your best not to overdo it.

So, in short, yes, you can have too much fiber. Considering that the general population is in a fiber deficit, this is a more rare problem. However, if you do have symptoms, then it is best to not ignore it. Too much fiber may not be detrimental but it definitely is uncomfortable. It will stop your body from working at its best, and if left for too long, it could lead to other problems. The goal is to be healthy and help our bodies to function optimally and not to be overly compulsive when adding certain foods and food groups into our diets.

Chapter 5: How to Do a Fiber Cleanse

The background is important but the execution is what really counts; this will determine whether you reap the full benefits of the fiber cleanse or not. We have discussed what the fiber cleanse is and the benefits of incorporating it into your diet; let's dive into the how-to of a fiber cleanse.

Actions to Incorporate in the Fiber Cleanse

Doing a fiber cleanse is not only about eating a good amount of fiber. There are other factors that will help your body along this journey. Coming from a broader approach will help you to add things to your daily life that will help you get more out of the fiber cleanse and help you see results quicker.

Drink Water

We all know that water is important to our body. In fact, our body is made up of about two-thirds water, so if we do not get enough water, we will end up feeling tired and dehydrated. Many sources suggest drinking eight glasses of water a day but the more correct estimation is about 91 to 125 fluid ounces of water per day (*Water and Digestion: What You Need to Know*, n.d.). That may seem like a lot but this includes the water you get from your food. Also, remember tea and coffee do count but you should be careful how much of this you drink since caffeine is known to dehydrate you.

If you are constantly getting less water than you should, consider water tracking. This can be done manually or on an app. The purpose of this is to make a note of how much water you are drinking throughout the day. Some apps will even remind you when to drink a glass of water so you can be sure of getting in the recommended amount of water. You may not need to do this forever, because once it becomes a habit, you will just drink water automatically.

If you are not keen on the extra admin of water tracking, then you will just have to be more conscious of drinking water throughout the day. Sometimes, we are not even aware that we are thirsty and mistake the feeling for hunger. A good way to counteract that is to have a glass of water before every meal and snack. If you are still hungry, then you can go ahead and eat, but if you were just thirsty, you have saved yourself from consuming the extra calories.

Fiber and water work together in the digestive system, so making sure you are getting some water in at every meal will be really good for your body. Fiber soaks up the liquids in your digestive system to help with the eliminating process. As the stool moves through the body, it ends up in the colon; here, the water is squeezed out so it can be conserved for the body. If there are not enough liquids, you might end up being constipated. Getting enough water in your system is vital for the eliminating process.

Exercise

Exercise is something many of us love to hate; we know it's good for us but many people struggle to get into it. If you need a little more motivation, then it is good to note that exercise can actually help your digestive system. When we exercise, our blood flow increases, and this extra circulation is good for our digestive system and bodies in general.

Regularly incorporating exercise into your life will result in a healthy gut and the overall strengthening of the digestive tract. There have been other studies that have concluded that increased exercise is linked to a reduction in cancer risk and has a positive effect on the gut microbiota (Rosario, 2019). There are also short-term benefits to exercising, such as alleviating cramps, gas, and constipation.

Exercise not only aids in the sending blood to the digestive tract but it also increases metabolism. Metabolism is the rate in which your body burns up food for energy; the higher your metabolism, the more calories you will burn even if you are in a sedentary state. This will aid in weight loss.

Some exercises will be more beneficial to the digestive system, so if you are unsure of what exercise you want to do, then consider what will be mentioned here. Increasing the blood flow to the organs aids the digestive system: running, cycling, swimming, and other aerobic or cardiovascular exercises accomplish this. They increase the heart rate, which in turn, speeds up blood flow and increases metabolism. If you don't like these types of exercises or are unable to do them for, consider doing stretching and yoga. Yoga is especially good for the digestive system and there are specific yoga programs for the digestive tract. A quick search on Google or YouTube will help you find something beneficial.

At the end of the day, any exercise will be helpful to you in some way, so start small and work your way up. Even a post-meal walk can help your body digest your food; a walk is not strenuous enough to cause cramps or anything like that after eating. Not moving your body enough can have negative effects on your digestive system and your well-being. Just 20 to 30 minutes of walking a day will already hold massive benefits for you.

You should also be aware of what you are eating before a workout. Eating the wrong foods or eating too much food before you exercise can have some negative side effects. Eating a big heavy meal and then immediately going to work out might lead to heartburn, bloating, and even some abdominal pain. Your body needs blood flow in order to digest food efficiently, and if we over exert ourselves when exercising, the blood moves away from the digestive tract and pumps towards the heart and the organs that are in use. Give yourself about one to two hours after eating before you engage in any intense activity.

Meals high in fats and proteins can be especially bad for you before exercise. If you are planning on getting a pre-workout snack, try and eat high fiber, high carbohydrate foods. These foods are more easily digestible and won't cause any gastrointestinal problems. Try eating bananas, oats, or whole wheat toast; these foods can actually be beneficial to your workout since it will give you the energy you need. To be safe, wait a few minutes before you start exercising after you eat these. Remember to drink lots of water; exercising is very dehydrating.

Introducing Fiber Into Your Diet

As you start switching your diet over to a more high fiber one, you might experience some discomfort and gas because your body is not used to it. This is why it is best to try and add it in slowly. Suddenly adding in a whole lot of fiber to your diet will cause your body to react badly.

The best way to go about it is to add in an extra serving of fiber per week. Start by replacing your white sandwich bread with whole wheat bread, then the next week add in a serving of fresh veggies to your lunch. Every week up your fiber intake a bit until you get to the recommended amount per day. This should ease your body into it.

Since gas can be a problem when you decide to change your diet, remove other food sources that cause gas. Sodas and gum are gas-causing snacks, so avoid them as much as possible so you do not suffer from excessive gas; once your body gets used to the new diet, you can add them in again. Every person is different, so there may be foods your body just doesn't agree with or that react and cause gas for you. Take note of these foods; perhaps keeping a food journal will help with this. Once you are aware of these foods, you can lower your intake until your body is used to the increased fiber.

Eating Both Types of Fiber

Both insoluble and soluble fiber are important to the digestive process, so you need to make sure you are getting both. They both perform slightly different actions but they work together in the body. Eating a variety of high fiber foods should help with that and many foods have both types of fiber in them.

In general, you pretty much eat any food that has fiber in it but if you want to specifically get either insoluble or soluble fiber into your diet, there are foods that are high in each. For insoluble fiber, try and eat foods that have a rougher texture, like whole wheat grains, couscous, green beans, spinach, kale, and root vegetable skins. Sources of soluble fiber are oats, lentils, nuts, apples, beans, and many other fruit and vegetables.

Getting a Balanced Diet

Having a good amount of fiber in your diet is important but you should be getting a balanced diet in all areas. When you are thinking of your meals, try and add in all the food groups and not a majority of high fiber carbohydrates. Fiber will help your body get the most out of all the other foods you are eating.

You still need protein and fats, so look at your meals holistically. White breads, pastas, and rice don't add much to your diet, so swapping them for their brown and whole wheat alternative is great, but make sure you also have a source of protein (lean meats, fish, legumes, nuts, and dairy) and some healthy fat (nuts, seeds, fish, and avocado). As you can see, some of the foods overlap, so if you plan your meals correctly, one type of food can check off many boxes.

Fiber Supplements

In general, there is nothing wrong with taking a fiber supplement if you are really struggling to get the fiber you need from food. Of course, the best way is always the natural way; the supplements do not have the nutrients and vitamins high fiber foods contain. If you are considering taking a fiber supplement, I would suggest you first try and add fiber in naturally through foods and then make that decision.

If you have any current health problems that are affecting your digestive system, like irritable bowel syndrome or Crohn's disease, then you will need to talk to your doctor before taking a fiber supplement. Fiber supplements are also known for blocking the effects of certain medications; Aspirin and Carbamazepine are examples of this. It can also drop blood sugar levels, so if you are diabetic, then you might have to adjust your insulin medication (Mayo Clinic, 2018b).

As with adding fiber into your diet, you will need to adjust to the fiber supplement. Try the smallest dosage first and then slowly increase it; this will give your body a chance to get used to it and may ease bloating and gas. The best thing you can do is increase your fiber intake as much as possible and then supplement the shortfall. This way you are not relying totally on the supplement and can still get some of the benefits from high fiber foods.

Probiotics and Fiber

Systems in our gut work together to make sure everything is running smoothly. When we eat fiber, the good bacteria in our gut love it; they feed off the fiber. This good bacteria help with the breakdown of food and keeps our gut healthy.

Sometimes, we do not have enough of these healthy gut bacteria and that is where probiotics come in. Probiotics are live healthy gut bacteria and they help balance your intestinal flora (Dean, n.d.). You can consume these probiotics via probiotic supplements or you can get it naturally through foods. Probiotic cultures can be found in foods such as yogurt and kefir; most manufacturers will label these foods stating that they have probiotic cultures in them.

Having these probiotics once a day will help the digestion of food and keep the gut happy. Since fiber and probiotics work together in the gut, increasing both of them will be very beneficial to digestive processes. However, probiotics do have the same effects as fiber in terms of gas and bloating. To reduce these symptoms, try and slowly introduce the probiotics into your diet.

What Daily Fiber Intake Might Look Like

As we have been discussing, it is important to get the right amount of fiber into your daily diet. We have discussed some foods that are high in fiber and even some food swaps you can do to easily incorporate fiber into your diet. However, we have not yet touched on what a healthy high-fiber diet actually looks like. That is the aim of this portion of the chapter; I want to provide you with a good picture of a high-fiber diet so you know what to do and what to look for in your daily meal planning. All of these meal plans fall between 25 and 35 grams of fiber per day. We have included three snack options; you do not have to eat three snacks a day if you are not hungry.

Example 1

Breakfast: A serving of whole grain bran cereal and milk, plus a small banana or half a large one.

Lunch: Turkey or ham sandwich (bread must be whole wheat). Add some lettuce and tomato and either an apple or orange on the side.

Dinner: Your choice of fish served with half a cup of spinach and half a cup of lentils. For a side, have a salad made with lettuce and carrots.

Snack 1: A handful of almonds (about 20 - 24) and a handful of raisins.

Snack 2: Yoghurt and half a cup of berries of choice.

Snack 3: A serving of home-popped popcorn.

Example 2:

Breakfast: Two boiled, poached, or scrambled eggs on top of two slices of whole wheat bread. Have a whole orange on the side.

Lunch: Baked potato with the skin, filled with 150 g of baked beans and 30 g of cheese. Add a leafy green salad on the side.

Dinner: Vegetable chili. Add in four or five of your favorite vegetables instead of meat to your chili recipe.

Snack 1: One cup of strawberries

Snack 2: 4 prunes

Snack 3: 4 whole wheat cracker and cheese

Example 3

Breakfast: Homemade or low sugar muesli with milk and an apple.

Lunch: A Waldorf salad.

Dinner: A chicken breast served with 100 g of potatoes and a side of broccoli.

Snack 1: A small handful of sunflower seeds and 3 dried apricots.

Snack 2: Peach slices and yoghurt; you can sprinkle some chopped almonds or chia seeds over top if you would like.

Snack 3: A small bowl of berries or grapes.

High Fiber Foods

To make it easier for you to plan and swap out different foods, have a look at the provided guide to see how much fiber can be found in high fiber foods. It will be easier to make sure you are getting the right amount of fiber if you are able to track what is in your food. Remember, for a female over 18 and under 50 years old, you should be getting about 25 grams of fiber per day, and for a male in the same age range, you should be getting 38 grams per day.

If you are buying packaged foods, check the label since that will give you the most accurate information. This is just a general estimate; weight, size, and other factors might change the amount of fiber in these foods. This information was taken from Mayo Clinic (2018a) and C.S Mott Children's Hospital (n.d.).

Fruit:

- 1 cup of raspberries - 8 g of fiber
- 1 medium pear - 5.5 g of fiber
- 1 medium apple - 4.5 g of fiber
- 1 medium banana - 3.0 g of fiber
- 1 medium orange - 3 g of fiber
- 1 cup of strawberries - 3 g of fiber
- 1 cup of blueberries - 4 g of fiber
- 10 prunes - 6 g of fiber
- ⅔ cup of raisins - 4 g of fiber

Vegetables, Nuts, and Seeds:

- 1 cup of boiled peas - 8 g of fiber
- 1 cup of broccoli - 5 g of fiber
- 1 cup of Brussels sprouts - 4 g of fiber

- 1 medium baked potato with the skin - 4 g of fiber
- 1 cup of sweet corn - 3.5 g of fiber
- 1 cup of baked beans - 14 g of fiber
- 1 cup of pinto beans - 14.7 g of fiber
- 1 cup of lima beans - 13.2 g of fiber
- ½ a cup of boiled spinach - 2.2 g of fiber
- 1 medium sweet potato - 3 g of fiber
- 1 cup of boiled lentils - 15.5 g of fiber
- 1 cup of boiled split peas - 16 g of fiber
- 1 ounce of chia seeds - 10 g of fiber
- 1 ounce of almonds - 3.5 g of fiber
- 1 ounce of sunflower seeds - 3 g of fiber

Cereals, Grains, and Breads:

- 1 cup of whole wheat spaghetti - 6 g of fiber
- 1 cup of barley - 6 g of fiber
- 1 cup of quinoa - 5 g of fiber
- 1 cup of oatmeal - 5 g of fiber
- 3 cups of popped popcorn - 3.5 g of fiber
- 1 cup of brown rice - 3.5 g of fiber
- 1 slice of whole wheat bread - 2 g of fiber
- 1 slice of rye bread - 2 g of fiber
- ½ a cup of All-Bran flakes - 10 g of fiber

Conclusion

Fiber is a very important part of a healthy digestive system and a healthy body in general. The two types of fiber, insoluble and soluble, work together to both collect everything that needs to be eliminated and then eliminate it smoothly. The fiber cleanse allows the body to clean itself; the body already has all the systems it needs but it does require some help.

It is never a good idea to eliminate an entire food group. Our bodies are designed to function by using the three major food groups; protein, fats, and carbohydrates. If we lack any of these, then we are depriving our bodies of something it needs. It is not about only adding in fiber and then forgetting everything else; it is important to remember that everything in our bodies work together in some way. The foods we put in will dictate how well our bodies are able to function. We should always be aiming for a healthy and well-balanced diet.

Getting these food groups are important but it is even more important to know where your nutrients are coming from. You need high-quality sources of food. Most foods that are high in fiber are high quality and they are natural. Natural, whole foods will always have more nutrients in them because they have not been refined. It is important to be aware of where your food is coming from and what is in the food you place in your body.

Remember that there are also other factors that play a part in a fiber cleanse; while what you put into your body is an important pillar, you also need to keep yourself hydrated and get enough exercise; these help with digestion and the general process of waste removal in the body.

The fiber cleanse will allow you to kick-start your health journey and really take care of your gut. The gut is so important because it helps you maintain your overall well-being with the gut bacteria assisting in fighting off sicknesses and sending signals to the brain to help regulate your hormones and nervous system (UC Davis Health, 2019). A well-balanced diet that includes a healthy amount of fiber is key to overall well-being.

References

Agatston, A. (2009, November 5). *Fiber and Heart Health - Heart Health - Everyday Health*. EverydayHealth.com. https://www.everydayhealth.com/heart-health-expert/fiber-and-heart-health.aspx

Bodian, C. H. (2019, March 8). *4 Positive Effects of Exercise on the Digestive System*. LIVESTRONG.COM. https://www.livestrong.com/article/356356-immediate-effects-of-exercise-in-the-digestive-system/

Brusie, C., & Cirino, E. (2017, April 18). *Can You Use Your Diet to Cleanse Your Colon?* Healthline. https://www.healthline.com/health/digestive-health/colon-cleanse-diet

Butler, N. (2017, August 17). *Soluble and insoluble fiber: Differences and benefits*. MedicalNewsToday. https://www.medicalnewstoday.com/articles/319176#soluble-vs-insoluble-fiber

Collins, K. (2018, September 21). *Ask The Dietitian: Get Your Facts Right on Fiber and Whole Grains*. American Institute for Cancer Research. https://www.aicr.org/resources/blog/ask-the-dietitian-get-your-facts-right-on-fiber-and-whole-grains/

Crusader. (2016, June 28). *7 Things That Can Happen When You Don't Get Enough Fiber*. Chicagocrusader.Com. https://chicagocrusader.com/7-things-can-happen-dont-get-enough-fiber/

C.S Mott Children's Hospital. (n.d.). *Fiber in Foods Chart*. https://www.med.umich.edu/mott/pdf/mott-fiber-chart.pdf

Dean, D. (n.d.). *Probiotics & Fiber Supplements*. LIVESTRONG.COM. https://www.livestrong.com/article/288419-probiotics-fiber-supplements/

Dreisbach, S. (n.d.). *10 Amazing Health Benefits of Eating More Fiber*. EatingWell. http://www.eatingwell.com/article/287742/10-amazing-health-benefits-of-eating-more-fiber/

Fries, W. C. (2007). *4 Warning Signs Your Diet May Lack Fiber*. WebMD. https://www.webmd.com/food-recipes/features/4-warning-signs-your-diet-may-lack-fiber#1

Harvard Health Publishing. (2013, August). *Rethinking fiber and hydration can lead to better colon health.* Harvard Health. https://www.health.harvard.edu/diseases-and-conditions/rethinking-fiber-and-hydration-can-lead-to-better-colon-health

Jennings, K. (2016, July 27). *16 Easy Ways to Eat More Fiber.* Healthline. https://www.healthline.com/nutrition/16-ways-to-eat-more-fiber#section11

Kellow, J. (n.d.). *High Fibre Diet Plan 7-Day Menu.* WeightLossResources.co.uk. https://www.weightlossresources.co.uk/diet/high_fibre/plan_sample.htm

Leiva, C. (2019, June 13). *10 dangers of a low-fiber diet, from constipation to colon cancer.* Insider. https://www.insider.com/dangers-of-a-low-fiber-diet-constipation-to-colon-cancer-2019-6

Matala, N. (2018, September 19). *Increase Fiber to Decrease Cholesterol.* Raleigh Medical Group. https://www.raleighmedicalgroup.com/blog/entryid/528/how-to-lower-cholesterol-with-fiber

Mayo Clinic. (2018a). *How much fiber is found in common foods?* Mayo Clinic. https://www.mayoclinic.org/healthy-lifestyle/nutrition-and-healthy-eating/in-depth/high-fiber-foods/art-20050948

Mayo Clinic. (2018b, October 25). *Should you take daily fiber supplements?* Mayo Clinic. https://www.mayoclinic.org/healthy-lifestyle/nutrition-and-healthy-eating/expert-answers/fiber-supplements/faq-20058513?reDate=23052020

Mayo Clinic. (2018c, November 16). *Dietary fiber: Essential for a healthy diet.* Mayo Clinic. https://www.mayoclinic.org/healthy-lifestyle/nutrition-and-healthy-eating/in-depth/fiber/art-20043983

McManus, K. D. (2019, February 21). *Should I be eating more fiber?* Harvard Health Blog. https://www.health.harvard.edu/blog/should-i-be-eating-more-fiber-2019022115927

Natural Cleanse vs Detox: The Benefits of High Fiber and Water. (2015, September 14). NuGo Fiber d'Lish. https://www.nugofiber.com/blog/water-fiber-better-than-juice-cleanse/

Olsen, N. (2018, March 22). *Too much fiber: Symptoms and treatment.* Medicalnewstoday. https://www.medicalnewstoday.com/articles/321286#symptoms

Rodriguez, D. (2011, September 13). *Getting Fiber Without Excessive Gas.* EverydayHealth.Com. https://www.everydayhealth.com/digestive-health/getting-fiber-without-excessive-gas.aspx

Rosario, E. (2019, July 25). *Boost your digestive health through exercise.* Copeman Healthcare Centre. https://www.copemanhealthcare.com/resources/digestive-health-exercise

Santos-Neves, C. (n.d.). *Adding Fiber To Your Diet.* Epicurious. Retrieved June 4, 2020, from https://www.epicurious.com/archive/healthy/news/fiber

Schneeman, B. O. (1999). *Building scientific consensus: the importance of dietary fiber.* The American Journal of Clinical Nutrition, 69(1), 1–1. https://doi.org/10.1093/ajcn/69.1.1

Szalay, J. (2015, August 27). *What Is Fiber?* Live Science. https://www.livescience.com/51998-dietary-fiber.html

UC Davis Health. (2019, July 22). *What is "gut health" and why is it important?* UC Davis Health Newsroom. https://health.ucdavis.edu/health-news/newsroom/what-is-gut-health-and-why-is-it-important/2019/07#:~:text=A%20healthy%20gut%20contains%20healthy

Water and Digestion: What You Need to Know. (n.d.). Www.Benefiber.Com. https://www.benefiber.com/fiber-in-your-life/fiber-and-wellness/water-and-digestion/

Zelman, K. M. (2011, February 3). *How to Eat 37 Grams of Fiber in a Day.* WebMD. https://www.webmd.com/diet/eat-this-fiber-chart